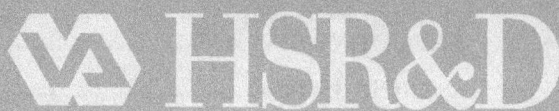

Comparative Effectiveness Review

Benign Prostatic Hyperplasia (BPH) Management in Primary Care – Screening and Therapy

Final Report
February 2007

Mark Helfand, MD, MPH, FACP
Staff Physician
Portland VA Medical Center
Portland, OR

Tara Muzyk, Pharm.D.
Clinical Pharmacist
VA Southern Nevada Healthcare System
Las Vegas, NV

Mark Garzotto, MD
Staff Physician, Urology Section
Portland VA Medical Center
Portland, OR

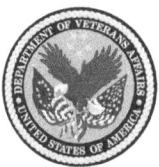

TABLE OF CONTENTS

EXECUTIVE SUMMARY

Background

Benign prostatic hyperplasia (BPH) causes urinary hesitancy and intermittency, weak urine stream, nocturia, frequency, urgency, and the sensation of incomplete bladder emptying. These symptoms, collectively called "lower urinary tract symptoms," or LUTS, can significantly reduce quality of life. Men with no symptoms or mild symptoms (AUA Symptom Index [SI] score of <7 points), and those who tolerate moderate symptoms well, may be managed without pharmacotherapy ("watchful waiting"). For those who have moderate or severe symptoms, medical treatments include alpha-1-selective adrenergic receptor (a-1-AR) antagonists, 5-alpha-reductase inhibitors (5-aRIs), or a combination therapy with one drug from each of these classes.

This report addresses the following questions about treatment for BPH:

1. For patients with BPH, what are the comparative benefits, harms, and efficacy of combination therapy with a 5-alpha-reductase inhibitor plus an alpha blocker versus either treatment alone?

2. What are the comparative efficacy and harms of alpha-1-adrenergic antagonists?

3. Are there subgroups of patients based on demographics (age, racial groups), other medications, or co-morbidities for which one treatment is more effective or associated with fewer adverse events?

Results

Combination therapy versus an alpha blocker or 5-ARI alone.

In the first year of treatment, alpha blockers are more effective than finasteride in improving symptoms. Combination therapy and an alpha blocker alone have similar effects on quality of life in the first year and a half of treatment.

For men who have BPH and have a large prostate or a high PSA at baseline, combination therapy can prevent about 2 episodes of clinical progression per 100 men per year over 4 years of treatment. There is no additional benefit within the first year of treatment. Most men who take combination therapy will have no additional benefit, and about 4 additional patients per 100 will become impotent who would not have taking an alpha blocker alone. Combination therapy can also be instituted after clinical progression occurs, but this strategy, while used widely, has not been studied.

There is considerable uncertainty about how best to monitor PSA in whom to choose to take finasteride or combination therapy and who are otherwise candidates for PSA screening. Candidates for combination therapy—patients who have large prostates and at least moderate symptoms—tend to have higher PSA levels than other patients who have BPH. Finasteride reduces prostate size and PSA levels, making detection of prostate cancer more difficult. Alpha-blockers do not affect PSA levels. Expanding access to combination therapy as an initial option would require higher utilization of ultrasound and PSA testing in BPH patients to assess the risk of progression. The consequences of such a program in a primary care setting have not been studied.

Choice of Alpha Blocker.

Previous, good-quality systematic reviews found that the alpha blockers, including alfuzosin prolonged-release and doxazosin GITS, have similar efficacy in improving symptoms and urinary flow rate. Observational studies of doxazosin, terazosin, and tamsulosin in selected patients indicate that in most patients who respond to an alpha blocker and who tolerate it well initially, the drug continues to work and to be well-tolerated for many years.

Head-to-head trials of alpha-blockers are few, small, and have serious limitations. They do not adequately test commonly held beliefs about differences in the side effect profiles of the alpha blockers. Specifically, they do not prove that, when used in practice, tamsulosin causes fewer cardiovascular adverse effects than other alpha-blockers because it does not reduce blood pressure. In placebo-controlled trials, tamsulosin caused higher rates of sexual ejaculation abnormalities than other alpha blockers. The placebo-controlled trials do not adequately test the hypothesis that use of tamsulosin as initial therapy reduces the risk of symptomatic hypotension.

For combination therapy, doxazosin is the best-studied alpha blocker.

Treatment of BPH in subgroups of patients.

Long-term observational studies establish that BPH can be treated safely with alpha blockers in patients taking other medications for hypertension. Alpha blockers should not be used as initial treatment for patients with hypertension, even those with BPH, because they are associated with poorer long-term outcomes than other choices. Data on the safety of alpha blockers in patients taking erectile dysfunction drugs are sparse.

Recently, the FDA issued a notice that intraoperative Floppy Iris Syndrome (IFIS) has been observed during phacoemulsification cataract surgery in some patients currently or recently treated with tamsulosin.

INTRODUCTION

Benign prostatic hyperplasia (BPH) causes urinary hesitancy and intermittency, weak urine stream, nocturia, frequency, urgency, and the sensation of incomplete bladder emptying. These symptoms, collectively called "lower urinary tract symptoms," or LUTS, can significantly reduce quality of life. Approximately 50% of men who have BPH develop moderate to severe symptoms. BPH is the 4th most commonly diagnosed disease among patients ≥50 years, after coronary disease and hyperlipidemia; hypertension; and type 2 diabetes. Among men over 50 years the prevalence of diagnosed BPH in the community is 13.5%.

Reducing symptoms is the main reason to treat BPH. Men with no symptoms or mild symptoms (AUA Symptom Index [SI] score of <7 points), and those who tolerate moderate symptoms well, may be managed without pharmacotherapy ("watchful waiting"). Medical treatments include alpha-1-selective adrenergic receptor (a-1-AR) antagonists, and 5-alpha-reductase inhibitors (5-aRIs).

Several reasons to choose one treatment instead of another have been suggested. A clinician may consider several factors in choosing a treatment:

- expeditious relief of the presenting symptoms and quality of life
- quality of life related to adverse effects of medications such as sexual dysfunction, dizziness, and asthenia
- preventing or delaying progression (especially acute urinary retention) in the long-term
- the risk of developing cancer
- the effect of treatment on hypertension, diabetes, post-traumatic stress disorder, and other conditions common among veterans.

Combination therapy with an alpha blocker plus a 5-aRIs, finasteride, has become increasingly popular [1, 2] since December, 2003, when the NIH-funded Medical Therapy of Prostatic Symptoms (MTOP) trial [3] was published. The trial found that the patients taking a combination of finasteride and doxazosin were less likely to develop acute urinary retention (AUR), an increase in symptom score greater than 4 points on the AUA/IPSS scale, or invasive therapy for BPH.

Wider use of combination therapy raises several issues for the VA:

1. Should the VA change its clinical practice guidelines to increase access to combination therapy?
2. Should the VA increase access to combination therapy by allowing primary care physicians to prescribe it?
3. How should patients taking finasteride or combination therapy be monitored for prostate cancer?

Current VA Guidance

In September, 2004, the VHA Pharmacy Benefits Management Strategic Healthcare Group and the Medical Advisory Panel published guidelines for the use of combination therapy. This guideline recommended combination therapy in two groups of patients: (A) those who had persistence or clinical progression of BPH symptoms while taking maximal doses of an alpha-blocker and (B) those who present with an AUA score ≥ 12 and have a prostate size >40 ml (see Figure 1). They did not offer specific guidance for PSA testing in patients taking finasteride, but some facilities recommend annual testing.

Figure 1. PBM-MAP Guidance on Combination Therapy.

Guidance on Combination Therapy with an Alpha-Blocker and Finasteride for BPH

A. Patients currently receiving monotherapy with an alpha-blocker at maintenance doses (e.g., doxazosin 8 mg qd, prazosin 4 mg BID, terazosin 10 mg qd, tamsulosin 0.4 mg qd or alfuzosin 10mg qd) or at highest tolerated dose if maintenance dose was not achieved, who have a large prostate (typically >40ml, or approximately the size of a golf ball)* and:

 ❑ Clinical progression of BPH symptoms as suggested by either:
  - An increase in the AUA symptom score ≥4 points from baseline
  - A history of acute urinary retention
    OR
 ❑ Persistently bothersome symptoms despite adequate alpha-blocker therapy, as above*

OR

B. Patients who have not tried alpha-blockers but have symptoms of benign prostatic hypertrophy who have a baseline AUA score of ≥12 and who are at high risk for an intervention or urinary retention because of a large prostate volume (typically >40ml, or approximately the size of a golf ball)*

*The risks and benefits of long-term finasteride therapy should be discussed with the patient. At this time finasteride is not recommended for prevention of prostate cancer based on the Prostate Cancer Prevention Trial. Patients should be reevaluated on a regular basis.

The PBM/MAP has also recommended against the addition of dutasteride and alfuzosin to the National VA Formulary.

AUA Guidelines

The American Urological Association published guidelines for management of BPH in 2003. It is described as having been updated in 2006, but it is not clear what material was updated. The AUA's main findings regarding the choice of drug therapies are:

- Alpha blockers are more effective than finasteride in improving symptoms
- Finasteride is not an appropriate treatment for patients who do not have prostate enlargement

- Finasteride is an appropriate treatment for patients who have LUTS and a large prostate
- The combination of an alpha-adrenergic receptor blocker and a 5 alpha-reductase inhibitor (combination therapy) is an appropriate and effective treatment for patients who have a high baseline risk of progression, but a specific threshold of risk cannot be determined.
- Alfuzosin, doxazosin, tamsulosin and terazosin have similar effectiveness
  - While side effect profiles differ, none of these drugs had a clear advantage as initial therapy.

The AUA guidelines also state that "Data are insufficient to support a recommendation for the use of prazosin." However, data on prazosin were not analyzed in developing the guidelines (page 3-13).

Advocates of wider use of combination therapy argue that "moderate to severely symptomatic patients with larger glands and higher serum PSA levels, however, are best served with combination therapy, as they benefit from the disease modification induced by the 5 alpha reductase inhibitors in addition to the symptomatic improvement due to the alpha blockers." [4] The AUA guidelines do not specify a threshold risk of progression above which combination therapy is the treatment of choice, but imply that there is such a threshold. Based on the guidance in Figure 1, in the VA combination therapy is an option for initial treatment in men who have at least moderate symptoms and a large prostate; however, within the VA there is no group for which combination therapy is described as the treatment of choice.

The purpose of this review is to compare finasteride in combination with an alpha-blocker to finasteride alone or to an alpha blocker alone, and to compare the efficacy and safety of different alpha-blockers (listed in Table 1). Combination therapy is used variably, within VHA. The balance of benefits and harms of finasteride, and its complex effects on detection of prostate cancer, and on the natural history of cancer, make it important that the VA implement evidence-based approach to treating BPH.

Table 1. Drug Indications and Dosing

Drug	Starting Dosage	Maintenance Dosage	On VA Formulary
Alfuzosin extended release	10 mg daily	10 mg qd	No
Doxazosin – Cardura®, generic	1 mg daily	2 to 8 mg daily	Yes
Doxazosin Gastro-Intestinal Therapeutic System	4 mg daily	8 mg qd	No
Prazosin	1 mg daily	2 to 10 mg	Yes
Tamsulosin – Flomax® (Boehringer Ingelheim)	0.4 mg daily	0.4 or 0.8 mg	No
Terazosin – Hytrin®, generic	1 mg daily	2 to 10 mg	Yes

Scope and Key Questions

Key Question 1: For patients with BPH, what are the comparative benefits, harms, and efficacy of combination therapy with a 5-alpha-reductase inhibitor plus an alpha blocker versus either treatment alone?

Key Question 2: what are the comparative efficacy and harms of alpha-1-adrenergic antagonists?

Key Question 3: Are there subgroups of patients based on demographics (age, racial groups), other medications, or co-morbidities for which one treatment is more effective or associated with fewer adverse events?

Eligibility Criteria

Population(s): Adult patients in outpatient settings with the following diagnosis:
1. Benign prostatic hyperplasia (BPH)
2. Lower urinary tract symptoms (LUTS)

Interventions
1. Terazosin
2. Doxazosin
3. Tamsulosin
4. Prazosin
5. Finasteride
6. Combination of an alpha blocker and a 5-alpha-reductase inhibitor

Efficacy outcomes
1. Reduction in BPH or LUTS symptoms
    o Improvement in maximum flow rate (Qmax)
    o Reduction in International Prostate Symptom Score (IPSS or AUA score)
    o Reduction in irritative or obstructive symptoms

2. Delaying progression to acute urinary retention, worsening symptoms, or invasive therapy

Safety and related outcomes
1. Adverse drug reactions
2. Withdrawals due to adverse drug reactions
3. Hypertension, hypotension, sexual dysfunction
4. detection of prostate cancer

Study designs
For efficacy outcomes
1. controlled clinical trials that directly compared 2 or more of the interventions listed above
2. systematic reviews
3. placebo-controlled trials if they addressed outcomes not adequately addressed in direct comparison studies

For safety outcomes
1. controlled clinical trials and good-quality systematic reviews
2. cohort studies of a defined population

Trials were excluded if they
- evaluated phytotherapeutic agents or drugs that are not available on the VA National Formulary
- were not available in English
- had less than 30 days of follow up

METHODS see Appendix.

RESULTS

Overview

Searches identified 10 relevant systematic reviews. [5-14] We also identified 41 articles reporting 7 observational studies relevant to Key Question 1, including 11 about the risk for progression of BPH; 12 about prostate cancer detection or the incidence of cancer on treatment; and 18 about the comparative efficacy and/or safety of combination therapy, finasteride alone, and an alpha blocker alone. For comparisons of different alpha blockers (Key Question 2), we relied on relevant systematic reviews, [6, 9-13] supplemented by trials and observational studies published since 2003. For Key Question 3, we identified 11 publications of the use of alpha blockers or finasteride in the elderly or in patients with comorbid conditions, most commonly hypertension. [14-24]

Key Question 1: For patients with BPH, what are the comparative benefits, harms, and efficacy of combination therapy with a 5-alpha-reductase inhibitor plus an alpha blocker versus either treatment alone?

In the first year of treatment, alpha blockers are more effective than finasteride in improving symptoms. [25] Alpha blockers are equally effective in relieving symptoms in men with large prostate glands and those with normal-sized prostate glands. [26, 27] Finasteride is more effective than placebo in relieving symptoms only in men with prostate size >40 cc and is less effective than an alpha blocker in the first year of therapy regardless of prostate size. [25, 28]

Because it has no advantage in the short-term, the main potential advantage of finasteride therapy or combination therapy is preventing or delaying progression of disease in the long-term. [29] Progression of BPH is usually defined as any of the following events: 1) an episode of acute, spontaneous urinary retention, 2) an increase in AUA symptom score of 4 or more points, or 3) surgery for BPH. Some definitions of progression include other events. For example, in the Veterans Affairs Cooperative Study of transurethral resection vs. watchful waiting in 591 veterans (mean AUA score 14.1), 47 patients (17%) in the watchful waiting group experienced treatment failure, defined as the occurrence of any of the following events during 3 years of follow-up: death; repeated or intractable urinary retention; a residual urinary volume over 350 ml; the development of a bladder calculus; new, persistent incontinence requiring the use of a pad, penile clamp, or condom; a symptom score of 24 or higher at one visit or scores of 21 or higher at two consecutive visits; or a doubling of the base-line serum creatinine concentration.[30] In the TUR group, 23/280 (8%) failed treatment.

In judging the need for finasteride or combination therapy, it is important to consider several factors:

- *How serious a threat to health and well-being are progression events?*
- *What is the risk of progression?*
- *By how much does finasteride or combination therapy reduce the risk?*
- *What are the risks and bother from side effects of finasteride or combination therapy?*

Smaller trials, and those with a duration of one year or less, accrue too few progression events to compare the longer term balance of benefits and risks of alpha-blocker therapy to finasteride alone or to combination therapy. For this reason, the evidence base for comparing combination therapy to single-drug therapy is limited to a few well-known trials. [3, 25, 31-33]

How serious is progression?
AUR or advancing symptoms cause significant expense and reduce the quality of life, but they are treatable conditions with a good prognosis. Most men who present with AUR will eventually require surgery, but transurethral resection as well as other effective treatment options are available for patients who progress.

What is the risk of progression?
Population-based cohort studies as well as the control groups of randomized trials of treatments for LUTS provide information about the risk of progression.

About 60% of first episodes of acute urinary retention (AUR) occur in men who have a diagnosis of BPH. Table 2 shows annual rates of AUR, symptom progression, and surgery for some large cohort studies and trials. The 2nd line of data from Olmsted County indicates that men in Olmsted County who met the inclusion criteria for the MTOPs trial had substantially higher rates of events than the MTOPs sample. [34] This result means that the MTOPS results may not represent results in other practice settings.

Table 2. Progression Events per 1,000 men.

Type of progression event →	Acute Urinary Retention	Symptom Progression	Surgery	All
Cohorts				
Health Professionals Study (AUA score 8-19)	11.1			
Health Professionals Study (AUA score >20)	14.3			
Olmsted County (all)	8.5	97	6.6	105
Olmsted County (similar to MTOPS)	18.3	86.5	16.8	109
Placebo groups				
MTOPS	6	36		45*
PREDICT	15	11		
PLESS	10		25	

Data from [29, 34] [35-37]
*Included UTI and incontinence.

Predicting the risk of progression.
Older age, prostate size, and PSA, high increasing symptom severity, a poor maximum urinary flow rate (Qmax), and a high post void residual urine volume (PVR) are established predictors of progression. [38, 39] Most studies of these risk factors, including analyses of the placebo groups of Proscar Long-Term Efficacy and Safety Study (PLESS)[40, 41] and MTOPs [42], confirm that the traditional risk factors are associated with progression, but fail to combine the factors into a sensitive, specific clinical prediction rule. In the "Olmsted County Study of Urinary Symptoms in Men" the relative risk of acute urinary retention in patients with prostate volumes >30 mL was three times greater than that in patients with a prostate volume of <30 mL. [38]

In the MTOPs trial, 128 of 737 men (17%) in the placebo group progressed over 4 years. [42] About 80% of the progression events were an increase in symptoms of 4 or more AUA points from baseline. A PSA$\geq$1.6 ng/mL was associated with a higher risk of progression. After 4 years, 22% of men who had a PSA$\geq$1.6 ng/mL vs. 12% of men who had a PSA<1.6 ng/mL progressed. This difference can be expressed as approximately 22 additional cases per 1000 men per year (52 vs. 30 per 1000 men each year). Higher prostate volume ($\geq$ 31 mL vs. <31 ml) lower Qmax ($\geq$ 10.6 mL/sec vs. <10.6 mL/s), and higher post-void residual volume ($\geq$39 mL vs. <39 mL) were also associated with progression.

Similarly, in PLESS, over 4 years 99 of 3,040 men (6.6%) experienced AUR. Half of these episodes of AUR were spontaneous; the others were precipitated by surgery or other interventions. The incidence of spontaneous acute urinary retention increased with increasing prostate volume divided into tertiles (14 to 41 mL; 42 to 57 mL; >57 mL) from 0% to 1.7% and 6.0%, respectively, over a 4-year period. [43] The incidence of combined, spontaneous, and precipitated acute urinary retention increased from 4.4% to 14.0%, from the smallest to the largest volume tertile. In the placebo-controlled finasteride trials generally, the 2-year incidence of spontaneous AUR was 4.2% in men with prostate volume>40 ml vs. 1.6% in the <40 ml group. [44] Higher baseline PSA was associated with a higher risk of progression, defined as acute urinary retention or the need for surgery. [43] A PSA≥3.2 ng/mL was associated with an 18% risk of progression, versus 12% for 1.4≤PSA<3.2 ng/mL and 7% for PSA<1.4 ng/dL.

It is not known whether the additional risk related to a higher PSA or prostate volume is additive, or whether there is a more complicated relationship among factors. In MTOPs, for example, higher prostate volume was not associated with age or baseline symptom scores, but was highly correlated with post-void residual and PSA results. [31] In fact, the risk for a patient who has none of these risk factors, or more than one of them, has not been reported. As noted in the AUA guidelines, the lack of a validated prediction rule makes it difficult to specify a threshold for initial treatment with combination therapy. [45]

By how much does finasteride or combination therapy reduce the risk of progression?

Characteristics of the subjects of the major long-term trials of combination therapy are summarized in **Table 3, Part 1.** The VA Cooperative trial and Prospective European Doxazosin and Combination Therapy (PREDICT) were well-designed, one-year trials. Both found that an alpha blocker was better than finasteride for relieving symptoms. [25, 32, 33]

Trials of Combination Therapy. Part 1. Design and Patient Characteristics.

Trial name (Pub Yr)	Alpha Blocker(s)	5-alpha-reductase inhibitor	Years of recruitment	Number of Subjects	Years of followup	Inclusion criteria					Placebo group			
						Age	AUA/IPSS scores	Symptom score	Prostate volume	PSA	Progression	Spontaneous Acute Urinary Retention	≥ 4pt. Increase in AUA score
								mean± SD	mean± SD	mean± SD	# per 1000/year	# per 1000/year	# per 1000/year
VA Cooperative (1996)	terazosin 10 mg/d	finasteride 5 mg/d	1992-1994	1229	1	45-80	8 or greater	15.8±5.5	38.4±1.3	2.4±2.1	------------no data------------		
PREDICT (2003)	doxazosin 8 mg/d	finasteride 5 mg/d		1095	1	50-80	12 or greater	17.2±4.5	36±14*	2.6±2.1	not reported	15	11
MTOPS (2003)	doxazosin 8 mg/d	finasteride 5 mg/d	1993-1998	3047	4.5	>50	8 or greater	16.8±5.9	35.2±18.8	2.3±2.0	45	6	36
PLESS (1998)	none	finasteride 5 mg/d		3040	4			15±6	55±26	2.8±2.1	32.5	10	NR
PROWESS (1998)	none	finasteride 5 mg/d		3270	2	50 to 75					30	13	NR
SMART (2003)	tamsulosin	dutasteride		327	0.7	>45	12 or greater						

* Estimated by DRE.

The Medical Therapy of Prostatic Symptoms trial was designed to test whether, with a longer follow up, finasteride and combination therapy, but not an alpha-blocker alone, would prevent or delay progression of BPH. [3] The mean patient age at randomization was 62.6 years (±7.3 years). Patients were Caucasian (82%), African American (9%), Hispanic (7%), Asian (1%) or Native American (<1%). The mean duration of BPH symptoms was 4.7 years (±4.6 years). Patients had moderate to severe BPH symptoms at baseline with a mean AUA symptom score of approximately 17 out of 35 points. Mean maximum urinary flow rate was 10.5 mL/sec (±2.6 mL/sec). The mean prostate volume as measured by transrectal ultrasound was 36.3 mL (±20.1 mL). Prostate volume was ≤20 mL in 16% of patients, ≥50 mL in 18% of patients and between 21 and 49 mL in 66% of patients.

The main results of MTOPs are shown in Table 3, Part 2. Overall, for every 22 patients treated with combination therapy instead of doxazosin alone, one instance of progression would be prevented over 4 years.

AUR. In the MTOPs trial, the cumulative incidence of acute urinary retention at 4 years in the finasteride and placebo groups was 0.8% and 2.4%, respectively, so if 100 men were treated for 4 years only 2 cases of AUR would be prevented. Alpha blockers alone do not appear to affect rates of AUR.

Recent meta-analyses of studies of finasteride vs. placebo provide the best available estimates of its effects on progression (Table). [5, 7] In PLESS, if 100 men were started on finasteride instead of placebo, by 4 years four men would avoid AUR. In the placebo controlled finasteride trials generally, in men who had a prostate size >40 ml, finasteride reduced the 2-year incidence of AUR from 4.2% to 1.8%. In men who had a prostate size <40 ml, the 2-year incidence in the placebo group was only 1.6%. [44] Similarly, finasteride reduced AUR incidence more in patients who had a PSA>1.4 ng/ml (from 3.9% to 1.6% over 2 years) than in those with a PSA<1.4 ng/ml (from 0.5% to 0.024%).

Symptomatic Progression.
About 75% of progression events are due to an increase in symptom score rather than a dramatic event such as AUR. Alpha blockers as well as finasteride reduce the risk of symptomatic progression. MTOPs found that doxazosin alone and finasteride alone reduced the risk of clinical progression to a similar degree, [3] but not as much as combination therapy. The event rates shown below, from MTOPs, reflect symptomatic progression rates. Compared with doxazosin alone, combination therapy prevented 1 symptomatic progression for every 20 patients treated for 4 years. (Conversely, 19 of 20 patients treated for 4 years did not benefit symptomatically from combination therapy.)

Surgery.
Among the major trials, and across time, rates of surgery vary widely, most likely due to practice styles rather than patient characteristics. In MTOPs, 26 (3%) of 756 patients assigned to doxazosin required invasive therapy by 4 years, versus 14 (2%) per 768 finasteride patients and 12 (1%) of 786 combination therapy patients.

Table 3. Part 2. With permission from Bandolier. [46]

	Placebo	Doxazosin		Finasteride		Combination	
Number of patients	737	756		768		786	
Outcome	Percent	Percent	NNT (95% CI)	Percent	NNT (95% CI)	Percent	NNT (95% CI)
Any clinical BPH progression	17	9.7	15 (10 to 27)	10	16 (10 to 34)	5.3	9 (7 to 12)
Symptom score increase ≥4 points	13	7.3	17 (11 to 35)	8.5	21 (13 to 64)	4.6	12 (9 to 17)
Acute retention	2.4	1.2	NS	0.8	60 (34 to 260)	0.5	52 (32 to 140)
Invasive BPH therapy	5.0	3.4	NS	1.8	31 (20 to 74)	1.5	27 (19 to 59)

MTOPS was reported in 2003, but results for subjects with different prostate gland sizes did not become available until early 2006. [31] Table 3, Part 2 compares the results of combination therapy in patients with a small, medium, or large gland. For men with a prostate size over 40 ml, *initial* therapy with finasteride plus doxazosin instead of doxazosin alone prevented one progression event for every 13 men treated for four years. It should be noted again that nearly 80% of these events were an increase in symptoms rather than less common, more serious events (AUR and invasive treatment).

Table 3, Part 3, Expected numbers of events per 1,000 men over 4 years by prostate size. Based on MTOPs. [31]

Prostate Size (percent of sample)*	All progression events			
	Doxazosin Alone	Finasteride Alone	Combination Therapy	NNT (Comb vs. Dox alone)
<25 ml (31%)	77	102	54	43
25 to 40 ml (28%)	**106**	102	**55**	20
>40 ml (31%)	**148**	147	**71**	13

*Total sample 3,047. **Bold=statistically significant for doxazosin vs. combination.**

Effect on Quality of Life.
After 16 months of treatment, combination therapy and an alpha blocker alone have similar effects on quality of life. (Figure, Copyright © 2003 American Urological Association Education and Research, Inc.)

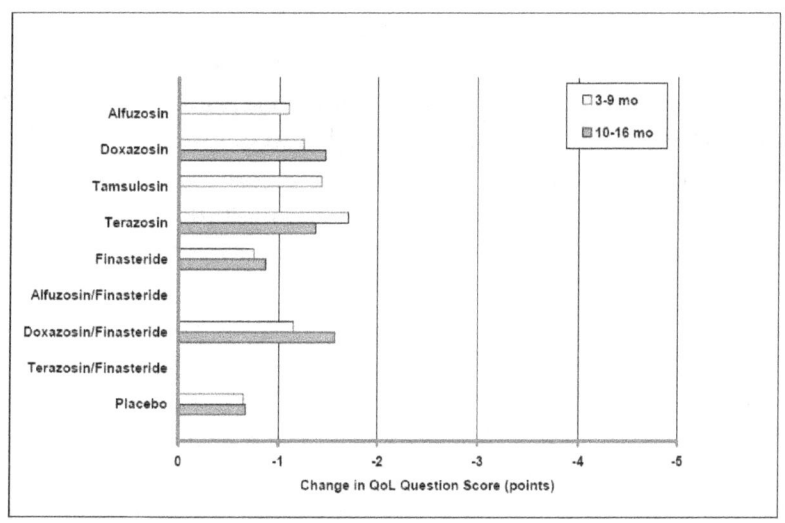

What are the risks of combination therapy (that is, of alpha blocker+finasteride) vs. alpha blocker alone?

Discontinuation rates in MTOPs were low relative to most other studies. Adverse event rates in MTOPs (Table 4) show that combination therapy caused a higher frequency of dizziness and sexual side effects than doxazosin alone, but was similar otherwise.

Table 4: Adverse events (% of men) in MTOPS over four years.
With permission from Bandolier. [46]

Adverse event	Placebo	Doxazosin	Finasteride	Combination
Discontinuation	--	27	24	18
Dizziness	2.3	4.4	2.3	5.4
Postural hypotension	2.3	4.0	2.6	4.3
Asthenia	2.1	4.1	1.6	4.2
Peripheral edema	0.7	0.9	0.7	1.3
Dyspnea	0.6	0.9	0.6	1.2
Erectile dysfunction	3.3	3.6	4.5	5.1
Decreased libido	1.4	1.6	2.4	2.5
Abnormal ejaculation	0.8	1.1	1.8	3.1

What other factors influence the balance of benefits and harms?

Risk of developing cancer
The Prostate Cancer Prevention Trial (PCPT) studied the long-term effect of finasteride on cancer rates. Other large, long-term prostate cancer prevention trials are currently in the enrollment phase, including the REDUCE trial, a study undertaken by GlaxoSmithKline involving the drug dutasteride. [47]

Patients recruited into the PCPT were expected to have a lifetime incidence of 16.7% and a rate of death from prostate cancer of 3% to 4%. In the PCPT finasteride decreased the 7-year period incidence of prostate cancer vs. placebo (18.4% vs. 24.4%), but high-grade (Gleason score 7-10) tumors were significantly more common in the finasteride group. [48] Put differently, over 7 years, for every 1000 patients, finasteride was associated with 7 fewer low-grade cancers, 61 fewer intermediate-grade cancers, 6 fewer ungraded cancers, and 14 additional high-grade ones for a net reduction of 61 cancers. (Finasteride does not have an FDA indication for chemoprophylaxis of prostate cancer.)

The meaning of these results has been debated extensively. A notable recent finding is that, over the course of the study, the rate of PSA increase for high-grade cancers was similar in finasteride-treated patients and in placebo-treated patients, suggesting the increase in high-grade cancers is likely to be real rather than artifactual. [49, 50] At any rate, even those experts who argue that this increase in high-grade tumors is artifactual agree that "the role of 5ARIs for prostate cancer chemoprevention needs further examination before it can be considered for wide recommendation." [51]

PSA Testing
There is considerable uncertainty about how best to monitor PSA in whom to choose to take finasteride or combination therapy and who are otherwise candidates for PSA screening. Candidates for combination therapy—patients who have large prostates and at least moderate symptoms—tend to have higher PSA levels than other patients who have BPH. Finasteride reduces prostate size and PSA levels, making detection of prostate cancer more difficult. Alpha-blockers do not affect PSA levels. [52]

The best strategy for monitoring is unclear. The "doubling" rule—performing a biopsy if twice the PSA level exceeds the threshold for biopsy—is a typical protocol. It is based on analysis of PSA data in the PLESS trial, which had four years of follow up and which found that the performance (sensitivity and specificity) of the doubled PSA for detecting prostate cancer in the finasteride patients was at least as good as the actual PSA level was in the placebo control group. [53]

New strategies, while based on a careful analysis of data from several trials, have not been applied in practice, and their influence on the frequency of biopsies or the overall detection of cancers is unknown. A new analysis of data from PLESS, PCPT, and trials of dutasteride found that PSA decreases gradually over the first year of treatment with finasteride.[54] Before one year of treatment has been completed, doubling the PSA can overestimate PSA, resulting in a high false positive rate and more biopsies. Because of the difficulty of interpreting PSA They recommended not obtaining biopsies until one year of therapy is complete. At that time and thereafter, instead of using an adjustment factor (such as doubling), a biopsy should be done when an annual PSA test is higher by 0.3 ng/ml or more than the lowest PSA level obtained during treatment (the nadir.) Alternatively , analysis of PSA data in the 7-year Prostate Cancer Prevention Trial (PCPT) suggests that the adjustment factor gradually increased from 2 (doubling) to 2.5 after 7 years of treatment. [49] During the trial, the PCPT finasteride arm was adjusted to 2.3 at study year 4 to try to achieve a rate of biopsies closer to that of the placebo group.

High utilization of tests
In primary care, the use of combination therapy as an initial treatment option would require routine

use of ultrasound to determine prostate size and PSA to identify men at high risk of progression. In current primary care practice, these tests are rarely if ever used to choose an initial therapy for BPH, although PSA is of course used frequently to screen for prostate cancer. An alternative approach would be to obtain only a PSA and, after appropriate screening for prostate cancer, offer men who have severe symptoms and a PSA level above 4 ng/mL combination therapy. This strategy—intended to avoid wider ultrasound testing in primary care—has not been examined in a formal study. For every 1000 patients with BPH seen in primary care, this approach would result in obtaining 1000 PSA tests to identify perhaps 70 candidates for combination therapy. Of these, if 50 accepted combination treatment, 10 would discontinue therapy (mostly because of adverse events), while treating the remaining 40 men for 4 years would prevent 4 episodes of progressive symptoms and 1 episode of acute urinary retention or invasive therapy.

How does a stepped approach compare with those of initial combination therapy?
As mentioned above, adding finasteride after progression has occurred on an alpha blocker is an alternative to initial treatment with combination therapy. The stepped approach has the advantage of avoiding finasteride therapy in those patients (approximately 19 of 20) who would not experience a benefit over four years compared with an alpha blocker alone.

Unfortunately, there is no evidence about the strategy of instituting combination therapy after progression occurs. Comparing the effectiveness of these different approaches in patients considered candidates for initial combination therapy might be a high priority for the VA.

Key Question 2: In head-to-head trials, for patients with benign prostatic hyperplasia (BPH), do the different alpha-1-adrenergic antagonists differ in efficacy or adverse events?

Previous, good-quality systematic reviews found that the alpha blockers, including alfuzosin prolonged-release and doxazosin GITS, have similar efficacy in improving symptoms and urinary flow rate. [5, 6, 9, 13] [10-12] The GITS formulation is not available at the VA.

The review articles primarily summarize placebo-controlled trials. This is because only a few head-to-head trials of different alpha-blockers have been done (Table 5). [55-60] The head-to-head studies ranged from 4 weeks to 3 months in duration. Four of the 5 studies were conducted in Asian men. These trials are summarized in Appendix 2 (Evidence Table).

Table 5. Head to head trials of alpha blockers.

	Doxazosin	Prazosin	Tamsulosin	Terazosin
Doxazosin	X	0	0	1
Prazosin			1	1
Tamsulosin				3
Terazosin				

Because they are few, small, and have serious limitations, the head-to-head trials do not adequately test commonly held beliefs about differences in the side effect profiles of the alpha blockers. Specifically, they do not prove that, when used in practice, tamsulosin causes fewer cardiovascular adverse effects than other alpha-blockers because it does not reduce blood pressure.

The most extensive meta-analysis comparing side effects of alpha-blockers in trials was conducted by the American Urological Association. Results of these analyses are shown in Table 6. Except for a higher rate of asthenia with doxazosin and a higher rate of sexual side effects with tamsulosin, none of the differences are statistically significant. More recent uncontrolled or placebo-controlled trials [22, 61, 62] do not change these findings.

Table 6. Meta-analysis of side effects of alpha blockers.

Outcomes of medical therapies: estimates of occurrence of adverse events

	Median Percentage (95% CI)								
	Acute Urinary Retention	Asthenia	Breast	Cardio-vascular	Cardio-vascular-Peripheral Edema	Cardio-vascular, Serious	Dizziness	GI Systems	Headache
Alpha Blockers									
Alfuzosin		4 (1-10)		1 (0-4)	0 (0-1)		5 (1-12)	10 (6-15)	5 (3-9
Doxazosin	0 (0-1)	15 (13-18)		2 (1-4)	1 (1-3)		13 (9-19)	10 (6-15)	8 (4-12)
Tamsulosin	4 (1-8)	7 (3-12)		8 (2-18)			12 (8-17)	11 (6-18)	12 (6-19)
Terazosin	4 (1-8)	12 (10-13)		2 (1-3)	4 (2-6)	0 (0-0)	15 (12-20)	5 (3-9)	7 (5-10)
Hormonal									
Finasteride	2 (1-2)	2 (1-4)	1 (0-2)	5 (2-10)		1 (0-3)	5 (2-10)	6 (3-10)	4 (2-6)
Combination									
Alfuzosin/finasteride	0 (0-1)	1 (0-2)				0 (0-1)	2 (1-4)		2 (1-3)
Doxazosin/finasteride	0 (0-1)	13 (9-17)		2 (1-4)			14 (11-19)	8 (6-12)	9 (6-13)
Terazosin/finasteride		14 (11-18)					21 (17-26)		5 (3-8)
Placebo	3 (2-5)	4 (3-5)	2 (0-5)	4 (2-7)	1 (1-2)	1 (1-1)	5 (4-7)	6 (4-9)	5 (4-7)

From AUA Guideline with permission. [45]

Table 6 (cont.). Meta-analysis of side effects of alpha blockers.

Outcomes of medical therapies: estimates of occurrence of adverse events (continued)

	Median Percentage (95% CI)							
	Hypotension Asymptomatic	Hypotension Symptomatic	Hypotension Symptomatic Postural	Hypotension Symptomatic Syncope	Respiratory-Nasal Congestion	Sexual-Ejaculation	Sexual-Erectile Problems	Sexual Libido
Alpha Blockers								
Alfuzosin		1 (0-3)		1 (0-3)	6 (1-15)		3 (1-6)	1 (0-4)
Doxazosin	5 (3-10)		4 (1-9)	0 (0-2)	8 (1-25)	0 (0-2)	4 (1-8)	3 (2-6)
Tamsulosin	7 (2-15)		3 (1-6)	1 (0-1)	11 (4-23)	10 (6-15)	4 (1-8)	
Terazosin	8 (2-18)	3 (1-8)	6 (3-11)	1 (1-3)	6 (4-10)	1 (1-2)	5 (3-8)	3 (1-5)
Hormonal								
Finasteride	4 (1-12)		2 (1-3)	1 (0-3)	9 (2-22)	4 (3-5)	8 (6-11)	5 (4-7)
Combination								
Alfuzosin/ finasteride	8 (6-11)		1 (0-2)			1 (0-2)	8 (5-11)	2 (1-4)
Doxazosin/ finasteride	3 (1-5)		3 (1-5)	2 (1-3)	18 (14-23)	3 (2-6)	10 (7-14)	3 (1-5)
Terazosin/ finasteride			9 (6-12)	2 (1-4)	10 (7-14)	7 (5-10)	9 (1-13)	5 (3-8)
Placebo	2 (1-3)	2 (0-5)	1 (1-2)	1 (0-1)	6 (3-10)	1 (1-1)	4 (3-5)	3 (3-4)

From AUA Guideline with permission. [45]

A limitation of the AUA analysis is that it did not separate out rates of side effects by dose. While all alpha blockers have higher rates of adverse effects at high doses, the increase is particularly marked for tamsulosin. In head-to-head trials, tamsulosin 0.2 mg had lower rates of withdrawal due to side effects than terazosin at various doses. [55, 56, 58, 60] Across trials of tamsulosin, however, the overall rate of withdrawals increased from 6.5% for tamsulosin 0.2 mg to 16.3% for tamsulosin 0.8 mg. [11] Similarly, "any adverse event" was reported by 5% of men receiving tamsulosin 0.2 mg and by 75% of men receiving tamsulosin 0.8 mg. [11] Rates of dizziness were 0% for 0.2 mg, 7% for 0.4 mg, and 18% for 0.8 mg. Tamsulosin is not available as 0.2 mg capsules in the United States.

Observational studies of doxazosin, terazosin, and tamsulosin in selected patients indicate that in most patients who respond to an alpha blocker and who tolerate it well initially, the drug continues to work and to be well-tolerated for many years. [63-68] [69]

Key Question 3: Are there subgroups of patients based on demographics (age, racial groups, and gender), other medications, or co-morbidities for which one treatment is more effective or associated with fewer adverse events?

Hypertension.
The one-year-long Hytrin Community Assessment Study is the largest, best-conducted evaluation the safety of an alpha blocker in patients with hypertension and BPH. [21] [70] In the trial, 555 of 2084 subjects had hypertension, some of whom were treated with other classes of medication. Terazosin lowered blood pressure significantly in untreated (by 5.3 mm Hg) and treated patients (6.7 mm Hg). It lowered blood pressure by about 12 mm Hg in patients who actually had high

blood pressure at baseline (that is, who were not adequately controlled on their other blood pressure medications). The incidences of blood pressure-related side effects in patients on terazosin were comparable between untreated (13.5%) and treated patients (14.3%), as were premature withdrawal rates, with 4.2% of untreated patients and 4.5% of treated patients withdrawing due to blood pressure-related side effects. Overall rates of side effects and of withdrawal due to side effects were similar in patients with and without hypertension. Terazosin may be less effective for BPH symptoms in patients who have uncontrolled hypertension than in normotensive or well-controlled patients,[23]but it is not yet clear whether terazosin differs from other alpha blockers in this respect.

Three long-term observational studies have evaluated the use of doxazosin in patients with hypertension. In two of these, doxazosin was used primarily to treat BPH but was also used as therapy for high blood pressure. [17, 18] In the other, ALLHAT, doxazosin was the primary treatment for hypertension in patients who did not have BPH. ALLHAT found that, compared with other choices for initial blood pressure control, doxazosin treatment resulted in a higher rate of heart failure among patients at risk for that condition. Probably no alpha blocker should be used as initial treatment for patients with hypertension who are at risk of developing heart failure.

We identified one long-term follow up study of tamsulosin that evaluated side effects in patients with various comorbidities. [71] The study had 19,365 patients identified through post-marketing surveillance. It found that tamsulosin was well tolerated in patients with hypertension and other conditions, but the study was confined to patients who had been on the medication for some time, so patients who had dropped out early because of side effects would have been missed.

Tadalafil, Vardenafil and sildenafil.
All alpha blockers can cause hypotension and priapism, raising concern that alpha blockers might cause serious side effects when administered with drugs for erectile dysfunction. Erectile dysfunction drugs and prazosin, terazosin, or alfuzosin should be given at least 4 hours apart. In a small (22 patient) placebo-controlled study of starting vardenafil in patients already taking tamsulosin 0.4 or 0.8 mg, 2 placebo patients and 1 vardenafil 10-mg patient had a drop of 20 mm Hg or more in standing DBP; and 1 vardenafil 10-mg patient had a standing SBP drop of 30 mm Hg or more; and 3 patients receiving vardenafil 20 mg/tamsulosin 0.4 mg reported dizziness. [16] While the authors concluded that combining the two drugs is safe, the sample is too small to be conclusive evidence that more serious adverse events would not occur in a larger study.

Cataracts.
Recently, the FDA issued a notice that intraoperative Floppy Iris Syndrome (IFIS) has been observed during phacoemulsification cataract surgery in some patients currently or recently treated with tamsulosin (Flomax®).

Age.
Finasteride appears to be equally effective in older and younger patients who have BPH. [15]

SUMMARY

For men who have BPH and have a large prostate or a high PSA at baseline, combination therapy can prevent about 2 episodes of clinical progression per 100 men per year over 4 years of treatment. There is no additional benefit within the first year of treatment. Most men who take combination therapy will have no additional benefit, and about 4 additional patients per 100 will become impotent who would not have taking an alpha blocker alone. Combination therapy can also be instituted after clinical progression occurs, but this strategy, while used widely, has not been studied.

Expanding access to combination therapy as an initial option would require higher utilization of ultrasound and PSA testing in BPH patients to assess the risk of progression. The consequences of such a program in a primary care setting has not been studied.

Alpha blockers have similar effectiveness and safety. For combination therapy, doxazosin is the best-studied alpha blocker.

REFERENCES

1. Fitzpatrick, J.M. and R.S. Kirby, *Two-drug therapy is best for symptomatic prostate enlargement: could a combination of doxazosin and finasteride change clinical practice?* BJU International, 2004. 93(7): p. 914-5.

2. McDonald, H., et al., *An economic evaluation of doxazosin, finasteride and combination therapy in the treatment of benign prostatic hyperplasia.* Canadian Journal of Urology, 2004. 11(4): p. 2327-40.

3. McConnell, J.D., et al., *The long-term effect of doxazosin, finasteride, and combination therapy on the clinical progression of benign prostatic hyperplasia.* New England Journal of Medicine, 2003. 349(25): p. 2387-98.

4. Roehrborn, C.G., *Drug treatment for LUTS and BPH: New is not always better.* European Urology, 2006. 49(1): p. 5-7.

5. *Benign Prostatic Hypertrophy: An update on drug therapy*, in *Therapeutics Letter*. 2006.

6. Clifford, G.M. and R.D. Farmer, *Medical therapy for benign prostatic hyperplasia: a review of the literature.* European Urology, 2000. 38(1): p. 2-19.

7. Edwards, J.E. and M.R. A., *Finasteride in the treatment of clinical benign prostatic hyperplasia: a systematic review of randomised trials.* BMC Urol, 2002. 2: p. 1–17.

8. Andersen, J., et al., *Finasteride significantly reduces acute urinary retention and need for surgery in patients with symptomatic benign prostatic hyperplasia.* Urology, 1997. 49: p. 839-845.

9. Milani, S. and B. Djavan, *Lower urinary tract symptoms suggestive of benign prostatic hyperplasia: latest update on alpha1-adrenoceptor antagonists.* BJU International, 2005. 95 (Suppl4): p. 29-36.

10. Wilt, T.J., W. Howe, and R. MacDonald, *Terazosin for treating symptomatic benign prostatic obstruction: a systematic review of efficacy and adverse effects.* BJU International, 2002. 89(3): p. 214-25.

11. Wilt, T.J., R. MacDonald, and D. Nelson, *Tamsulosin for treating lower urinary tract symptoms compatible with benign prostatic obstruction: a systematic review of efficacy and adverse effects.* Cochrane Database of Systematic Reviews, 2002(4).

12. MacDonald, R., T.J. Wilt, and R.W. Howe, *Doxazosin for treating lower urinary tract symptoms compatible with benign prostatic obstruction: a systematic review of efficacy and adverse effects.* BJU International, 2004. 94(9): p. 1263-70.

13. Djavan, B. and M. Marberger, *A Meta-Analysis on the Efficacy and Tolerability of alpha1-Adrenoceptor Antagonists in Patients with Lower Urinary Tract Symptoms Suggestive of Benign Prostatic Obstruction.* Eur Urol 1999. 36: p. 1-13.

14. Barendrecht, M.M., et al., *Treatment of lower urinary tract symptoms suggestive of benign prostatic hyperplasia: the cardiovascular system.* BJU International, 2005. 95 Suppl 4: p. 19-28.

15. Kaplan, S.A., et al., *Comparison of the efficacy and safety of finasteride in older versus younger men with benign prostatic hyperplasia.* Urology, 2001 57: p. 1073-7.

16. Auerbach, S.M., et al., *Simultaneous administration of vardenafil and tamsulosin does not induce clinically significant hypotension in patients with benign prostatic hyperplasia.* Urology, 2004. 64(5): p. 998-1003; discussion 1003-4.

17. Fawzy, A., et al., *Long-term (4 year) efficacy and tolerability of doxazosin for the treatment of concurrent benign prostatic hyperplasia and hypertension.* International Journal of Urology, 1999. 6(7): p. 346-54.

18. Guthrie, R.M. and R.L. Siegel, *A multicenter, community-based study of doxazosin in the treatment of concomitant hypertension and symptomatic benign prostatic hyperplasia: the Hypertension and BPH Intervention Trial (HABIT).* Clinical Therapeutics, 1999. 21(10): p. 1732-48.

19. Kirby, R.S., *Terazosin in benign prostatic hyperplasia: effects on blood pressure in normotensive and hypertensive men.* British Journal of Urology, 1998. 82(3): p. 373-9.

20. Lowe, F.C., *Coadministration of tamsulosin and three antihypertensive agents in patients with benign prostatic hyperplasia: pharmacodynamic effect.* Clinical Therapeutics, 1997. 19(4): p. 730-42.

21. Lowe, F.C., P.J. Olson, and R.J. Padley, *Effects of terazosin therapy on blood pressure in men with benign prostatic hyperplasia concurrently treated with other antihypertensive medications.* Urology, 1999. 54(1): p. 81-5.

22. Muzzonigro, G., *Tamsulosin in the treatment of LUTS/BPH: an Italian multicentre trial.* Archivio Italiano di Urologia, Andrologia, 2005. 77(1): p. 13-7.

23. Sugaya, K., et al., *Influence of hypertension on lower urinary tract symptoms in benign prostatic hyperplasia.* International Journal of Urology, 2003. 10(11): p. 569-74; discussion 575.

24. Suzuki, H., *Treatment of benign prostatic hyperplasia and hypertension in elderly hypertensive patients.* British Journal of Urology, 1998. 81 Suppl 1: p. 51-5.

25. Lepor, H., et al., *The impact of medical therapy on bother due to symptoms, quality of life and global outcome, and factors predicting response. Veterans Affairs Cooperative Studies Benign Prostatic Hyperplasia Study Group.* Journal of Urology, 1998. 160(4): p. 1358-67.

26. Becopoulos, T., D. Mitropoulos, and I. Christofis, *Influence of prostate size on terazosin efficacy.* International Journal of Urology, 1997. 4(4): p. 358-61.

27. Boyle, P., et al., *Meta-analysis of randomized trials of terazosin in the treatment of benign prostatic hyperplasia.* Urology, 2001. 58(5): p. 717-22.

28. Boyle, P., A.L. Gould, and C. Roehrborn, *Prostate volume predicts outcome of treatment of benign prostatic hyperplasia with finasteride: meta-analysis of randomized clinical trials.* Urology, 1996. 48: p. 398-405.

29. McConnell, J.D., et al., *The effect of finasteride on the risk of acute urinary retention and the need for surgical treatment among men with benign prostatic hyperplasia. Finasteride Long-Term Efficacy and Safety Study Group.* N Engl J Med. , 1998 338: p. 557-63.

30. Wasson, J.H., D. Reda, J, and R.C. Bruskewitz, *A comparison of transurethal surgery with watchful waiting for moderate symptoms of benign prostatic hyperplasia.* N Engl J Med., 1995. 332: p. 75-79.

31. Kaplan, S.A., et al., *Combination therapy with doxazosin and finasteride for benign prostatic hyperplasia in patients with lower urinary tract symptoms and a baseline total prostatic volume of 25 Ml or greater.* Journal of Urology, 2006. 175: p. 217-21.

32. Lepor, H., et al., *The efficacy of terazosin, finasteride, or both in benign prostatic hyperplasia. Veterans Affairs Cooperative Studies Benign Prostatic Hyperplasia Study Group.* New England Journal of Medicine, 1996. 335(8): p. 533-9.

33. Kirby, R.S., et al., *Efficacy and tolerability of doxazosin and finasteride, alone or in combination, in treatment of symptomatic benign prostatic hyperplasia: the Prospective European Doxazosin and Combination Therapy (PREDICT) trial.[see comment].* Urology, 2003. 61(1): p. 119-26.

34.   Roberts, R.O., et al., *Limitations of using outcomes in the placebo arm of a clinical trial of benign prostatic hyperplasia to quantify those in the community.* Mayo Clinic Proceedings, 2005. 80(6): p. 759-64.

35.   Meigs, J.B., et al., *Incidence rates and risk factors for acute urinary retention: the Health Professionals Followup Study.* Journal of Urology, 1999. 162: p. 376-82.

36.   Roehrborn, C., et al., *Urinary retention in patients with BPH treated with finasteride or placebo over 4 years. The PLESS study group.* European Urology, 2000. 37(5): p. 528-36.

37.   Roehrborn, C.G., *Reporting of acute urinary retention in BPH treatment trials: importance of patient follow-up after discontinuation and case definitions.* Urology, 2002. 59(6): p. 811-5.

38.   Jacobsen, S.J., C.J. Girman, and M.M. Lieber, *Natural history of benign prostatic hyperplasia.* Urology, 2001. 58(6 Suppl 1): p. 5-16; discussion 16.

39.   Hong, S.J., et al., *Identification of baseline clinical factors which predict medical treatment failure of benign prostatic hyperplasia: an observational cohort study.* European Urology, 2003. 44(1): p. 94-9; discussion 99-100.

40.   Roehrborn, C.G., et al., *Storage (irritative) and voiding (obstructive) symptoms as predictors of benign prostatic hyperplasia progression and related outcomes.* European Urology, 2002. 42: p. 1-6.

41.   Roehrborn, C.G., et al., *Clinical predictors of spontaneous acute urinary retention in men with LUTS and clinical BPH: A comprehensive analysis of the pooled placebo groups of several large clinical trials.* Urology, 2001. 58: p. 210-6.

42.   Crawford, E.D., et al., *Baseline factors as predictors of clinical progression of benign prostatic hyperplasia in men treated with placebo.* Journal of Urology, 2006. 175(4): p. 1422-6; discussion 1426-7.

43.   Roehrborn, C., et al., *Serum prostate-specific antigen concentrations are a powerful predictor of acute urinary retention and need for surgery in men with clinical benign prostatic hypertrophy.* Urology, 1999. 53: p. 473-80.

44.   Marberger, M., et al., *Prostate volume and serum prostate-specific antigen as predictors of acute urinary retention.* European Urology, 2000. 38: p. 563-8.

45.   Roehrborn, C., et al., *AUA Guideline on the management of benign prostatic hyperplasia. American Urological Association Education and Research, Inc., (2003). Updated 2006 <http://auanet.org/guidelines/bph.cfm>. (10/28/04).* 2006.

46.   Bandolier, *Long-term BPH treatment.* 2004.

47.   Andriole, G., et al., *Chemoprevention of prostate cancer in men at high risk: rationale and design of the reduction by dutasteride of prostate cancer events (REDUCE) trial.* J Urol:, 2004. 172: p. 1314.

48.   Thompson, I., et al., *The influence of finasteride on the development of prostate cancer.* New England Journal of Medicine, 2003. 349: p. 215-224.

49.   Etzioni, R.D., et al., *Long-term effects of finasteride on prostate specific antigen levels: results from the prostate cancer prevention trial.* J Urol:, 2005. 174(3): p. 877-81. .

50.   Walsh, P.C., *Re: Long-term effects of finasteride on prostate specific antigen levels: results from the Prostate Cancer Prevention Trial.[comment].* Journal of Urology, 2006. 176(1): p. 409-10; author reply 410.

51.   Andriole, G., et al., *The effects of 5alpha-reductase inhibitors on the natural history, detection and grading of prostate cancer: current state of knowledge.* Journal of Urology, 2005. 174(6): p. 2098-104.

52. Roehrborn, C.G., et al., *Serial prostate-specific antigen measurements in men with clinically benign prostatic hyperplasia during a 12-month placebo-controlled study with terazosin. HYCAT Investigator Group. Hytrin Community Assessment Trial.* Urology, 1997. 50(4): p. 556-61.

53. Andriole, G.L., et al., *Treatment with finasteride preserves usefulness of prostate-specific antigen in the detection of prostate cancer: results of a randomized, double-blind, placebo controlled clinical trial. PLESS Study Group. Proscar Long-Term Efficacy and Safety Study.* Urology, 1998. 52: p. 195.

54. Marks, L.S., et al., *The Interpretation of Serum Prostate Specific Antigen in Men Receiving 5[alpha]-Reductase Inhibitors: A Review and Clinical Recommendations.* The Journal of Urology, 2006. 176(3): p. 868-874.

55. Lee, E. and C. Lee, *Clinical comparison of selective and non-selective alpha 1A-adrenoreceptor antagonists in benign prostatic hyperplasia: studies on tamsulosin in a fixed dose and terazosin in increasing doses.* British Journal of Urology, 1997. 80(4): p. 606-11.

56. Na, Y.J., Y.L. Guo, and F.L. Gu, *Clinical comparison of selective and non-selective alpha 1A-adrenoceptor antagonists for bladder outlet obstruction associated with benign prostatic hyperplasia: studies on tamsulosin and terazosin in Chinese patients. The Chinese Tamsulosin Study Group.* Journal of Medicine, 1998. 29(5-6): p. 289-304.

57. Narayan, P., M.P. O'Leary, and G. Davidai, *Early efficacy of tamsulosin versus terazosin in the treatment of men with benign prostatic hyperplasia: a randomized, open-label trial.* . J Appl Res, 2005. 5: p. 237-245.

58. Okada, H., et al., *A comparative study of terazosin and tamsulosin for symptomatic benign prostatic hyperplasia in Japanese patients.* BJU International, 2000. 85(6): p. 676-81.

59. Samli, M.M. and C. Dincel, *Terazosin and doxazosin in the treatment of BPH: results of a randomized study with crossover in non-responders.* Urologia Internationalis, 2004. 73(2): p. 125-9.

60. Tsujii, T., *Comparison of prazosin, terazosin and tamsulosin in the treatment of symptomatic benign prostatic hyperplasia: a short-term open, randomized multicenter study. BPH Medical Therapy Study Group. Benign prostatic hyperplasia.* International Journal of Urology, 2000. 7(6): p. 199-205.

61. Flannery, M.T., et al., *Efficacy and safety of tamsulosin for benign prostatic hyperplasia: clinical experience in the primary care setting.* Current Medical Research & Opinion, 2006. 22(4): p. 721-30.

62. Chung, B.H., S.J. Hong, and M.S. Lee, *Doxazosin for benign prostatic hyperplasia: an open-label, baseline-controlled study in Korean general practice.* International Journal of Urology, 2005. 12(2): p. 159-65.

63. Narayan, P., C.P. Evans, and T. Moon, *Long-term safety and efficacy of tamsulosin for the treatment of lower urinary tract symptoms associated with benign prostatic hyperplasia.* Journal of Urology, 2003. 170(2 Pt 1): p. 498-502.

64. Narayan, P. and H. Lepor, *Long-term, open-label, phase III multicenter study of tamsulosin in benign prostatic hyperplasia.* Urology, 2001. 57(3): p. 466-70.

65. Dutkiewicz, S., *Long-term treatment with doxazosin in men with benign prostatic hyperplasia: 10-year follow-up.* International Urology & Nephrology, 2004. 36(2): p. 169-73.

66. Ichioka, K., et al., *Long-term treatment outcome of tamsulosin for benign prostatic hyperplasia.* International Journal of Urology, 2004. 11(10): p. 870-5.

67.   Palacio, A., et al., *Long-term study to assess the efficacy of tamsulosin in the control of symptoms and complications developed in patients with symptomatic benign prostatic hyperplasia (OMNICONTROL study): first-year follow-up report.* Archivos Espanoles de Urologia, 2004. 57(4): p. 451-60.

68.   Schulman, C.C., et al., *Tamsulosin: 3-year long-term efficacy and safety in patients with lower urinary tract symptoms suggestive of benign prostatic obstruction: analysis of a European, multinational, multicenter, open-label study. European Tamsulosin Study Group.* European Urology, 1999. 36(6): p. 609-20.

69.   Lepor, H., *Long-term evaluation of tamsulosin in benign prostatic hyperplasia: placebo-controlled, double-blind extension of phase III trial. Tamsulosin Investigator Group.* Urology, 1998. 51(6): p. 901-6.

70.   Roehrborn, C.G., et al., *The Hytrin Community Assessment Trial study: a one-year study of terazosin versus placebo in the treatment of men with symptomatic benign prostatic hyperplasia. HYCAT Investigator Group.* Urology, 1996. 47(2): p. 159-68.

71.   Michel, M.C., et al., *Tamsulosin treatment of 19,365 patients with lower urinary tract symptoms: does co-morbidity alter tolerability?* J Urol:, 1998. 160: p. 784-91.

APPENDIX A: Methods for Evidence Synthesis

Literature Search

To identify relevant citations, we searched Ovid MEDLINE (1966 to July 2006.) For Key Question #1 we used the following search strategy:

1. exp Adrenergic alpha-Antagonists/ad, ae, cl, tu, ct, du [Administration & Dosage, Adverse Effects, Classification, Therapeutic Use, Contraindications, Diagnostic Use]
2. exp Prostatic Hyperplasia/mo, cl, co, di, pc, dh, dt, ep, su, th, ge [Mortality, Classification, Complications, Diagnosis, Prevention & Control, Diet Therapy, Drug Therapy, Epidemiology, Surgery, Therapy, Genetics]
3. 1 and 2
4. limit 3 (humans and male and "all adult (19 plus years)" and (clinical trial, phase i or clinical trial, phase ii or clinical trial, phase iii or clinical trial, phase iv or clinical trial or controlled clinical trial or evaluation studies or multicenter study or randomized controlled trial or technical report))
5. explode Finasteride
6. 3 and 5

For Key Questions #2 and #3, we used steps 1 to 4 of the same search string. We searched the Cochrane Database of Systematic Reviews (2nd quarter, 2006) but did not identify any additional systematic reviews.

All citations were imported into an electronic database (EndNote 9.0).

Study Selection

One reviewer assessed abstracts of citations identified from literature searches for inclusion, using the criteria described above. Full-text articles of potentially relevant abstracts were retrieved and a second review for inclusion was conducted by reapplying the inclusion criteria.

Data Abstraction

The following data were abstracted from included trials: study design, setting, population characteristics (including sex, age, ethnicity, diagnosis), eligibility and exclusion criteria, interventions (dose and duration), comparisons, numbers screened, eligible, enrolled, and lost to follow-up, method of outcome ascertainment, and results for each outcome. We recorded intention-to-treat results when reported. In cases where only per-protocol results were reported, we calculated intention-to-treat results if the data for these calculations were available. In trials with crossover, outcomes for the first intervention were recorded if available. This was because of the potential for differential withdrawal prior to crossover biasing subsequent results and the possibility of either a "carryover effect" (from the first treatment) in studies without a washout period, or "rebound" effect from withdrawal of the first intervention.

Data abstracted from observational studies included design, eligibility criteria duration, interventions, concomitant medication, assessment techniques, age, gender, ethnicity, number of patients screened, eligible, enrolled, withdrawn, or lost to follow-up, number analyzed, and results.

Quality Assessment

We assessed the internal validity (quality) of trials based on the predefined criteria listed in Appendix B. These criteria are based on the U.S. Preventive Services Task Force and the National Health Service Centre for Reviews and Dissemination (U.K.) criteria.[22, 23] We rated the internal validity of each trial based on the methods used for randomization, allocation concealment, and blinding; the similarity of compared groups at baseline; maintenance of comparable groups; adequate reporting of dropouts, attrition, crossover, adherence, and contamination; loss to follow-up; and the use of intention-to-treat analysis. Trials that had a fatal flaw in one or more categories were rated "poor-quality"; trials that met all criteria were rated "good-quality"; the remainder were rated "fair-quality." A fatal flaw occurs when there is evidence of bias or confounding in the trial, for example when randomization and concealment of allocation of random order are not reported and baseline characteristics differ significantly between the groups. In this case, randomization has apparently failed and for one reason or another bias has been introduced.

As the fair-quality category is broad, studies with this rating vary in their strengths and weaknesses: the results of some fair-quality studies are *likely* to be valid, while others are only *probably* valid. Those studies considered only *probably* valid are indicated as such using a "fair-poor" rating. A poor-quality trial is not valid—the results are at least as likely to reflect flaws in the study design as the true difference between the compared drugs. External validity of trials was assessed based on whether the publication adequately described the study population, how similar patients were to the target population in whom the intervention will be applied, and whether the treatment received by the control group was reasonably representative of standard practice. We also recorded the role of the funding source.

Appendix B also shows the criteria we used to rate observational studies. These criteria reflect aspects of the study design that are particularly important for assessing adverse event rates. We rated observational studies as good-quality for adverse event assessment if they adequately met six or more of the seven predefined criteria, fair-quality if they met three to five criteria and poor-quality if they met two or fewer criteria.

Included systematic reviews were also rated for quality based on pre-defined criteria (see Appendix B), based on a clear statement of the questions(s), inclusion criteria, adequacy of search strategy, validity assessment and adequacy of detail provided for included studies, and appropriateness of the methods of synthesis.

Overall quality ratings for the individual study were based on internal and external validity ratings for that trial. A particular randomized trial might receive two different ratings: one for effectiveness and another for adverse events. The overall strength of evidence for a particular key question reflects the quality, consistency, and power of the set of studies relevant to the question.

Evidence Synthesis

An evidence report pays particular attention to the generalizability of efficacy studies performed in controlled or academic settings. Efficacy studies provide the best information about how a drug performs in a controlled setting that allow for better control over potential confounding factors and bias. However, efficacy studies have some limitations, as the results are not always applicable to many, or to most, patients seen in everyday practice. This is because most efficacy studies use strict eligibility criteria which may exclude patients based on their age, sex, medication compliance, or severity of illness. For many drug classes severely impaired patients are often excluded from trials. Often, efficacy studies also exclude patients who have "comorbid" diseases, meaning diseases other than the one under study. Efficacy studies may also use dosing regimens and follow up protocols that may be impractical in other practice settings. They often restrict options, such as combining therapies or switching drugs, that are of value in actual practice. They often examine the short-term effects of drugs that, in practice, are used for much longer periods of time. Finally, they tend to use objective measures of effect that do not capture all of the benefits and harms of a drug or do not reflect the outcomes that are most important to patients and their families.

Data Presentation

We constructed evidence tables showing the study characteristics, quality ratings, and results for all included studies. Studies that evaluated one macrolide against another provided direct evidence of comparative benefits and harms. Outcomes of changes in symptom measured using scales or tools with good validity and reliability are preferred over scales or tools with low validity/reliability or no reports of validity/reliability testing. Where possible, head-to-head data are the primary focus of the synthesis. No meta-analyses were conducted in this review due to heterogeneity in treatment regimens, use of concomitant medications, outcome reporting and patient populations.

In theory, trials that compare these drugs to other interventions or placebos can also provide evidence about effectiveness. This is known as an indirect comparison and can be difficult to interpret for a number of reasons, primarily issues of heterogeneity between trial populations, interventions, and assessment of outcomes. Indirect data are used to support direct comparisons, where they exist, and are also used as the primary comparison where no direct comparisons exist. Such indirect comparisons should be interpreted with caution.

Appendix B: Trials comparing alpha antagonists

Clinical Trial	Inclusion Criteria/Pt. Population	Intervention	Results	Safety/Comments
Cam et al 2003 Prospective clinical study 178 patients doxazosin 4 mg 24 months no financial disclosure Turkish	Men > 50 years old IPSS 18-35 Attendance to a urology department due to: -LUTS -age > 50 -unremarkable medical hx in terms of LUTS -no definitive need for surgery	Doxazosin 1 mg titrated to 4 mg	Reduction in symptom scores from 24 (SD ±7.4) before medication to 17 (SD ±8.4) after 3 months of treatment In the patients reporting doxazosin as ineffective, no change, or effective, 93%, 59% and 15% respectively underwent surgery. Of the 178 patients enrolled 47% underwent surgery.	Evaluation of the efficacy doxazosin was determined by one multiple choice question regarding the satisfaction with the medical treatment in terms of relieving symptoms
Ichioka et al 2004 Prospective 123 patients 43 months Tamsulosin (n = 123) No financial disclosure Japanese	Men 53-88 years old Dx BPH Treated with tamsulosin >12 months	Tamsulosin 0.2 mg titrated up to 0.4 mg as needed to relieve sx.	Predictive for treatment failure: baseline IPSS ≥15, months 0-12 lowest IPSS ≥ 13, lowest QoL score of ≥ 3 and lowest BPH impact score of ≥ 4.	
Roehrborn et al 1996 Prospective, placebo controlled, randomized, double-blinded 2084 patients 1 year (Terazosin n = 1053 Placebo n = 1031) Funding: Abbot Labratorie American	Men ≥ 55 years old Moderate-severe BPH AUA-Symptom Score (SS) ≥ 13 AUA-Bother Score (BS) ≥ 8 PUF ≤ 15 mL/sec. Voided volume = 150 mL	Terazosin 1 mg x 3 days, 2 mg x 25 days, ↑ 5 mg or 10 mg as tolerated Placebo	Statistically superior improvements were observed in regard to AUA-BS, BPH impact index and the QoL score on terazosin-treated patients. PUF improved Treatment failure was higher in placebo	Withdraw was higher due to ADR was higher in terazosin patients

Study	Condition	Medication	Results	Adverse Effects
Okada et al 2000 Single-blind, randomized 61 patients 4 weeks Japanese	Symptomatic BPH	Terazosin 1-2 mg Tamsulosin 0.2 mg	Both meds significantly improved the total IPSS, irritative and obstructive symptom score, and quality of life. There was no significant difference for these variables between groups. There was no significant improvements between groups.	Incidence of ADR was not significantly different between groups. Neither medication affected systolic or diastolic blood pressure.
Lee et al 1997 Single-blind 98 patients randomized 8 weeks Korean	Moderate to severe BPH	Tamsulosin 0.2 mg Terazosin 1 mg ↑ 5 mg	Both medications similarly improved IPSS and Increased Qmax	Terazosin: -systolic and diastolic BP decreased significantly -dizziness, dry mouth were more frequent
Tsuiji et al 2000 Open-label 105 patietns Randomized (Prazosin n= 32, Terazosin n=35, Tamsulosin n=38) 4 weeks	LUTS associated with BPH	Prazosin 1 mg ↑ 2 mg Terazosin 1 mg ↑ 2 mg Tamsulosin 0.1 mg ↑ 0.2 mg	All significantly reduced subjective symptom scores from baseline. Terazosin significantly better improvement than Tamsulosin in 4 of 9 symptom scores (urgency, sense of residual urine, prolonged micturition, intermittency) Significant increase in flow with prazosin	ADR which lead to withdrawal: Prazosin = 1 Terazosin = 3 Tamsulosin = 0
Na et al 1998 Single-blinded, randomized 212 Patients Randomized 4 weeks Chinese	BPH	Terazosin 2 mg Tamsulosin 0.2 mg	Tamsulosin and terazosin: significant improvement in IPSS, Qmax and average urinary flow rate from baseline	Dizziness, hypotension occurred significantly more frequently with terazosin than tamsulosin

www.ingramcontent.com/pod-product-compliance
Lightning Source LLC
Chambersburg PA
CBHW081414170526
45166CB00010B/3342